Sculpting the Core: A Comprehensive Guide to Achieving Six-Pack Abs

Introduction:

In an era where fitness is not just a trend but a way of life, the quest for the elusive six-pack abs stands as a symbol of dedication, discipline, and determination. The allure of a sculpted midsection transcends mere aesthetics; it represents strength, health, and vitality. However, achieving this pinnacle of physical fitness requires more than just desire—it demands knowledge, strategy, and unwavering commitment.

"Sculpting the Core" is a comprehensive guide meticulously crafted to lead you through every step of the journey toward achieving six-pack abs. Whether you're a fitness novice or a seasoned athlete, this book is your roadmap to realizing your dream physique and unlocking the full potential of your core muscles.

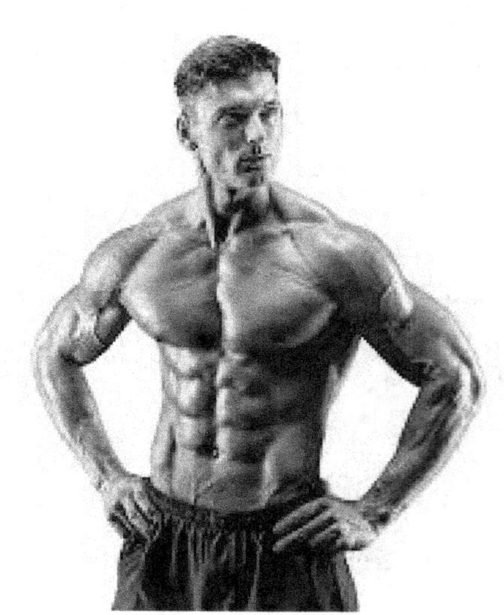

Chapter 1: Understanding the Core

- Defining the core: beyond just the abs
- Anatomy of the core: muscles involved and their functions
- The importance of core strength for overall fitness and performance

Chapter 2: Setting Your Goals

- Defining your objectives: aesthetics vs. functional strength
- Establishing realistic timelines and expectations
- The psychological aspect of goal setting and motivation

Chapter 3: Nutrition Essentials

- The role of nutrition in achieving visible abs
- Understanding macronutrients and their impact on body composition
- Crafting a personalized nutrition plan for optimal results

Chapter 4: Effective Workout Strategies

- The myth of spot reduction: debunking misconceptions
- Building a balanced workout routine: incorporating strength training, cardio, and flexibility
- Targeting the core: exercises for sculpting the abs, obliques, and lower back

Chapter 5: Mastering Core Exercises

- Core exercises for beginners, intermediate, and advanced levels
- Proper form and technique: maximizing effectiveness while minimizing injury risk
- Incorporating variety and progression for continuous improvement

Chapter 6: Supplementing Your Efforts

- The role of supplements in supporting your fitness goals
- Key supplements for enhancing fat loss and muscle development
- Safety considerations and potential risks associated with supplement use

Chapter 7: Overcoming Challenges

- Dealing with setbacks and plateaus: strategies for staying motivated
- Managing stress and its impact on fitness progress
- Cultivating a resilient mindset for long-term success

Chapter 8: Lifestyle Integration

- The importance of recovery: sleep, hydration, and stress management
- Incorporating fitness into daily life: making sustainable lifestyle changes
- Finding balance and enjoying the journey

Chapter 9: Navigating Plateaus and Adjustments

- Identifying signs of plateau and when to change your approach
- Adjusting your workout routine and nutrition plan for continued progress
- The role of rest and recovery in breaking through plateaus

Chapter 10: Celebrating Success and Sustaining Progress

- Recognizing milestones and celebrating achievements
- Strategies for maintaining your hard-earned results
- Embracing fitness as a lifelong journey

Conclusion:

"Sculpting the Core" is more than just a guidebook—it's a companion on your quest for six-pack abs and a healthier, stronger you. By equipping you with knowledge, strategies, and practical advice, this book empowers you to take control of your fitness journey and achieve results that transcend the physical. Embrace the process, stay committed, and let your transformed core become a testament to your dedication and perseverance.

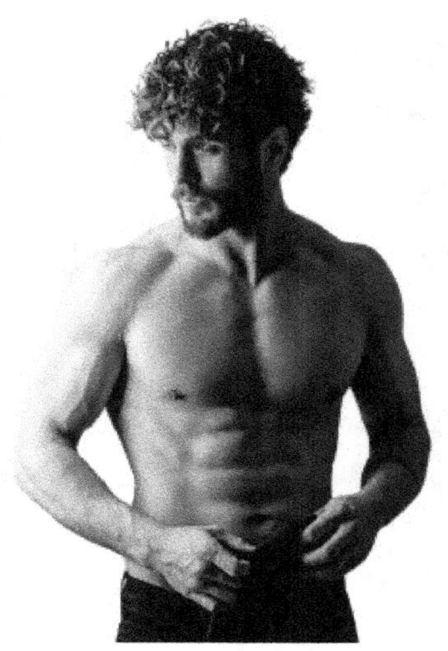

here's a sample six-pack abs workout plan. Remember to combine this routine with a balanced diet and sufficient rest for optimal results.

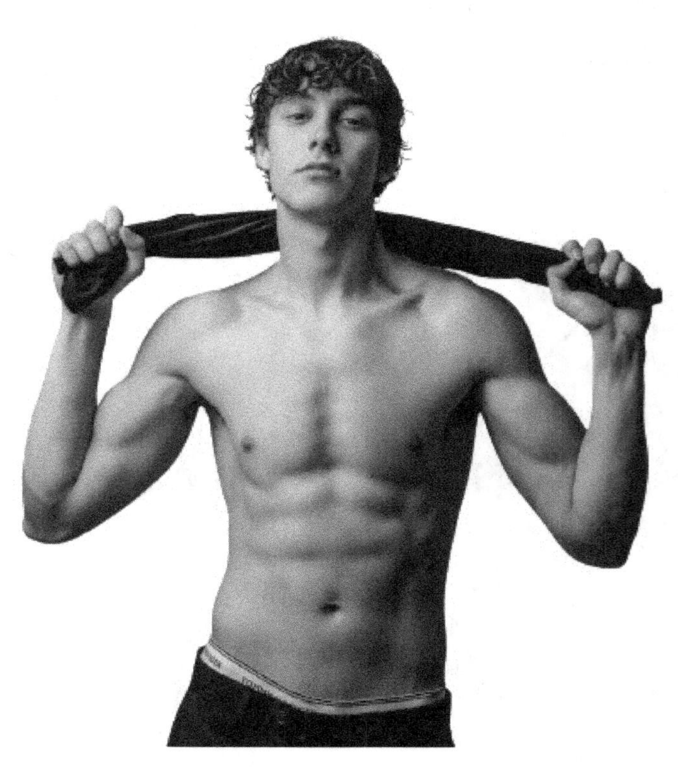

Day 1: Upper Abs

Crunches: 3 sets of 15 reps

Bicycle Crunches: 3 sets of 20 reps (10 each side)

Russian Twists: 3 sets of 15 reps (with or without weight)

Plank: 3 sets, hold for 30-60 seconds each

Leg Raises: 3 sets of 12 reps

Day 2: Lower Abs

Reverse Crunches: 3 sets of 15 reps

Hanging Leg Raises: 3 sets of 12 reps

Mountain Climbers: 3 sets of 20 reps (10 each leg)

Lying Leg Raises: 3 sets of 15 reps

Plank with Leg Lifts: 3 sets, hold for 30-45 seconds each

Day 3: Rest or Active Recovery

Engage in light cardio, yoga, or stretching to aid recovery.

Day 4: Obliques

Side Plank: 3 sets, hold for 30-45 seconds each side

Side Crunches: 3 sets of 15 reps (each side)

Woodchoppers: 3 sets of 12 reps (each side)

Russian Twists with Medicine Ball: 3 sets of 15 reps (each side)

Bicycle Crunches: 3 sets of 20 reps (10 each side)

Day 5: Full Abs

Plank to Push-Up: 3 sets of 10 reps

Spiderman Plank: 3 sets of 12 reps (each side)

Hanging Knee Raises: 3 sets of 12 reps

Cable Crunches: 3 sets of 15 reps

Swiss Ball Jackknife: 3 sets of 12 reps

Day 6: HIIT Cardio

Engage in high-intensity interval training (HIIT) to torch fat and reveal those abs!

Day 7: Rest

Allow your muscles to recover and grow.

Remember to adjust the number of sets and reps according to your fitness level and gradually increase intensity as you progress. Consistency is key, so stick to your routine and watch those six-pack abs take shape!

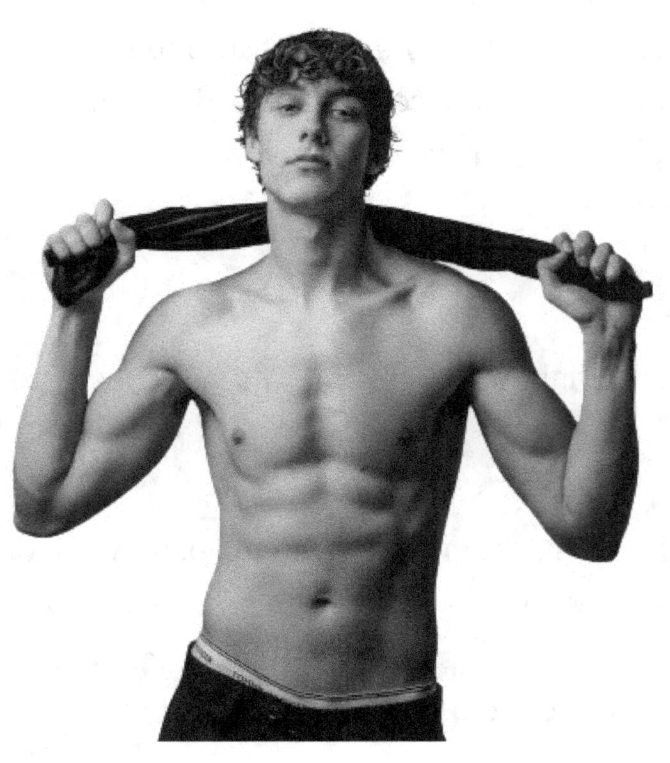

Chapter 1: Understanding the Core

In the pursuit of six-pack abs, it's essential to grasp the fundamentals of the core—a term that extends far beyond the visible abdominal muscles. This chapter delves into the intricacies of the core, from its definition to its significance in enhancing overall fitness and performance.

1.1 Defining the Core: Beyond Just the Abs

The core encompasses a complex network of muscles, ligaments, and tendons that provide stability and support to the spine and pelvis. While the rectus abdominis—the coveted "six-pack" muscles—often steal the spotlight, they represent only a fraction of the core. True core strength involves the coordinated activation of multiple muscle groups to maintain posture, transfer force, and facilitate movement.

Beyond the rectus abdominis, the core includes:

Transverse abdominis: The deepest abdominal muscle, responsible for compressing the abdomen and stabilizing the spine.

Internal and external obliques: Muscles located on the sides of the abdomen, aiding in rotation and lateral flexion of the trunk.

Erector spinae: Muscles along the spine that support spinal extension and maintain posture.

Multifidus: Deep muscles of the spine that stabilize individual vertebrae and assist in spinal stability.

Pelvic floor muscles: Muscles at the base of the pelvis, crucial for urinary and fecal continence, as well as providing support to the organs in the pelvis.

Diaphragm: The primary muscle involved in breathing, contributing to core stability through its connection to the transverse abdominis and pelvic floor.

Understanding the holistic nature of the core is essential for developing a comprehensive training regimen that addresses all its components, not just the superficial abdominal muscles.

1.2 Anatomy of the Core: Muscles Involved and Their Functions

To comprehend the core's role in movement and stability, it's crucial to explore the anatomy of its constituent muscles and their functions:

Rectus Abdominis: Located along the front of the abdomen, the rectus abdominis assists in trunk flexion and provides support for the internal organs.

Transverse Abdominis: Wrapping around the abdomen like a corset, the transverse abdominis stabilizes the spine and pelvis, serving as the body's natural weight belt.

Internal and External Obliques: These muscles facilitate trunk rotation and lateral bending, contributing to dynamic core stability and rotational power.

Erector Spinae: Comprising the iliocostalis, longissimus, and spinalis muscles, the erector spinae group supports spinal extension and maintains upright posture.

Multifidus: Deep within the spine, the multifidus muscles stabilize individual vertebrae, providing segmental support and contributing to spinal alignment.

Pelvic Floor Muscles: Including the pubococcygeus, iliococcygeus, and puborectalis muscles, the pelvic floor supports pelvic organs and assists in bladder and bowel control.

Diaphragm: As the primary muscle of respiration, the diaphragm contracts and relaxes to facilitate breathing while also contributing to core stability by coordinating with the transverse abdominis and pelvic floor muscles.

By understanding the specific roles of each core muscle, individuals can tailor their training to address weaknesses, improve functional movement patterns, and enhance overall core strength.

1.3 The Importance of Core Strength for Overall Fitness and Performance

Core strength serves as the foundation for nearly every movement the body performs, whether in daily activities or athletic pursuits. A strong core not only improves posture and spinal alignment but also enhances athletic performance, reduces the risk of injury, and enhances functional movement patterns.

Key benefits of a well-developed core include:

Improved Posture: Core muscles work synergistically to support the spine and pelvis, promoting proper alignment and reducing the risk of postural imbalances and related discomfort.

Enhanced Stability and Balance: Core stability is essential for maintaining equilibrium during static and dynamic movements, preventing falls, and improving balance in various activities.

Injury Prevention: A strong core provides a stable base for limb movement, reducing the risk of injuries to the spine, hips, and lower extremities during sports and physical activities.

Functional Strength: Core strength translates into improved performance in functional movements such as lifting, carrying, pushing, and pulling, enhancing overall physical capabilities.

Power Generation: The core acts as a transfer station for force generated by the lower body, efficiently transferring energy to the upper extremities during activities such as throwing, punching, and swinging.

Spinal Support and Health: Strong core muscles support the spine and help distribute forces evenly, reducing the risk of degenerative conditions such as disc herniation and spinal instability.

Incorporating core-specific exercises into a comprehensive fitness routine is essential for cultivating a robust core, optimizing athletic performance, and promoting long-term musculoskeletal health.

Understanding the core's multifaceted nature, anatomical components, and functional significance lays the groundwork for effective training strategies aimed at achieving six-pack abs and overall core strength. In the chapters that follow, we'll delve deeper into practical techniques, exercises, and principles for sculpting a strong, defined core that not only looks impressive but also enhances your quality of life and athletic performance.

Chapter 2: Setting Your Goals

In the pursuit of six-pack abs, setting clear and realistic goals is paramount to success. This chapter guides you through the process of defining your objectives, establishing achievable timelines, and tapping into the psychological aspects of goal setting and motivation.

2.1 Defining Your Objectives: Aesthetics vs. Functional Strength

Before embarking on your journey to sculpted abs, it's essential to clarify your primary objectives. Are you primarily focused on achieving aesthetic goals, such as visible six-pack abs and a lean physique? Or do you seek functional strength and core stability to enhance athletic performance and daily activities?

Aesthetics:

Seeking visible abdominal definition and a sculpted midsection.

Prioritizing exercises and nutrition strategies aimed at reducing body fat percentage and revealing muscle definition.

Emphasizing symmetry, proportion, and muscularity in pursuit of a visually pleasing physique.

Functional Strength:

Prioritizing core stability, balance, and functional movement patterns.

Focusing on exercises that improve overall core strength and dynamic stability, benefiting athletic performance and injury prevention.

Balancing aesthetics with performance-based goals to cultivate a strong, functional physique.

Understanding your primary objectives allows you to tailor your training and nutrition strategies accordingly, ensuring that your efforts align with your desired outcomes.

2.2 Establishing Realistic Timelines and Expectations

Achieving six-pack abs requires time, dedication, and consistency. Setting realistic timelines and managing expectations are crucial for maintaining motivation and sustaining long-term progress.

Consider the following factors when establishing timelines and expectations:

Current Body Composition: Assess your starting point in terms of body fat percentage, muscle mass, and overall fitness level. Realize that individuals with higher body fat percentages may take longer to achieve visible abdominal definition.

Rate of Progress: Understand that progress may vary from person to person based on factors such as genetics, metabolism, and adherence to training and nutrition protocols.

Sustainable Practices: Aim for gradual, sustainable progress rather than quick fixes or extreme measures. Sustainable habits lead to lasting results and minimize the risk of rebound weight gain or burnout.

Patience and Persistence: Recognize that achieving six-pack abs is a journey marked by ups and downs. Stay patient, trust the process, and remain committed to your goals, even in the face of challenges or setbacks.

By setting realistic timelines and managing expectations, you can avoid frustration and maintain motivation throughout your fitness journey.

2.3 The Psychological Aspect of Goal Setting and Motivation

The journey to six-pack abs is not solely physical—it also requires mental fortitude, resilience, and motivation. Understanding the psychological aspects of goal setting and motivation can empower you to overcome obstacles and stay focused on your objectives.

Key psychological factors to consider include:

Intrinsic vs. Extrinsic Motivation: Identify your internal reasons for pursuing six-pack abs, such as improved self-confidence, health, or personal fulfillment. While external motivators like social validation or competition may provide temporary boosts, intrinsic motivation sustains long-term commitment.

Goal Visualization: Visualize your desired outcomes, imagining yourself with sculpted abs and envisioning the benefits of achieving your fitness goals. Use visualization techniques to reinforce motivation and maintain focus during challenging times.

Positive Self-Talk: Cultivate a positive mindset by challenging self-limiting beliefs and replacing negative self-talk with affirmations and encouragement. Believing in your ability to succeed enhances resilience and fosters a growth-oriented mindset.

Accountability and Support: Surround yourself with a supportive community of friends, family, or fitness professionals who can offer encouragement, accountability, and guidance along your journey. Sharing your goals and progress with others enhances motivation and accountability.

By addressing the psychological aspects of goal setting and motivation, you can harness the power of your mind to propel you toward your fitness goals with confidence and determination.

Chapter 3: Nutrition Essentials

Nutrition plays a crucial role in achieving visible abs, shaping body composition, and optimizing overall health and performance. In this chapter, we'll explore the significance of nutrition in your quest for six-pack abs, delve into the role of macronutrients, and provide guidance on crafting a personalized nutrition plan tailored to your goals and preferences.

3.1 The Role of Nutrition in Achieving Visible Abs

While exercise is essential for building muscle and burning calories, nutrition is the cornerstone of achieving visible abs. A well-balanced diet provides the necessary nutrients to support muscle growth, reduce body fat percentage, and reveal the underlying abdominal muscles. Here's how nutrition impacts your journey to six-pack abs:

Caloric Balance: Achieving a caloric deficit—consuming fewer calories than you expend—is key to shedding excess body fat and revealing abdominal definition. However, it's crucial to strike a balance between calorie restriction and adequate nutrition to support muscle retention and overall health.

Macronutrient Distribution: Manipulating the proportion of macronutrients—protein, carbohydrates, and fats—in your diet influences body composition and energy levels. Prioritizing high-quality sources of protein, complex carbohydrates, and healthy fats supports muscle recovery, satiety, and metabolic health.

Nutrient Timing: Timing your meals and snacks strategically can optimize energy levels, enhance workout performance, and support muscle growth and recovery. Prioritizing nutrient-dense foods around workouts and spacing meals evenly throughout the day can help regulate hunger, stabilize blood sugar levels, and promote fat loss.

Hydration: Adequate hydration is essential for cellular function, digestion, and metabolism. Drinking plenty of water throughout the day helps maintain hydration levels, supports exercise performance, and may aid in appetite control and weight management.

Micronutrient Intake: In addition to macronutrients, micronutrients—vitamins, minerals, and antioxidants—are vital for overall health and optimal functioning of the body. Consuming a diverse array of fruits, vegetables, whole grains, and lean proteins ensures sufficient micronutrient intake and supports immune function, recovery, and vitality.

By prioritizing nutrient-dense foods, managing portion sizes, and maintaining a balanced diet, you can create the nutritional foundation necessary for achieving visible abs and sustaining long-term health and fitness.

3.2 Understanding Macronutrients and Their Impact on Body Composition

Macronutrients—protein, carbohydrates, and fats—serve as the building blocks of nutrition, each playing a distinct role in body composition, energy metabolism, and overall health. Understanding the impact of macronutrients can empower you to optimize your dietary intake for your physique goals.

Protein: As the primary building block of muscle tissue, protein is essential for muscle repair, growth, and maintenance. Consuming an adequate amount of protein supports muscle retention during periods of calorie restriction, promotes satiety, and enhances metabolic rate through the thermic effect of food. Aim to include lean protein sources such as chicken, turkey, fish, tofu, eggs, and legumes in each meal to support muscle development and recovery.

Carbohydrates: Carbohydrates serve as the body's primary source of energy, fueling workouts and supporting exercise performance. While low-carb diets may promote initial weight loss, carbohydrates are essential for replenishing glycogen stores, preserving muscle mass, and sustaining energy levels during intense training sessions. Focus on consuming complex carbohydrates such as whole grains, fruits, vegetables, and legumes, which provide sustained energy, fiber, and essential nutrients.

Fats: Despite their often-misunderstood reputation, dietary fats are crucial for hormone production, cellular function, and nutrient absorption. Incorporating healthy fats such as avocados, nuts, seeds, olive oil, and fatty fish into your diet supports satiety, enhances flavor and texture, and may have anti-inflammatory and cardiovascular benefits. Aim to include a balance of monounsaturated, polyunsaturated, and omega-3 fatty acids in your diet to promote overall health and optimize body composition.

Balancing your macronutrient intake according to your individual needs, activity level, and goals is essential for achieving and maintaining visible abs while supporting overall health and performance.

3.3 Crafting a Personalized Nutrition Plan for Optimal Results

Crafting a personalized nutrition plan tailored to your goals, preferences, and lifestyle is essential for achieving sustainable results and maximizing the effectiveness of your fitness regimen. Here's how to create a nutrition plan optimized for sculpting six-pack abs:

Assess Your Current Diet: Begin by evaluating your current dietary habits, including your typical food choices, portion sizes, meal timing, and nutrient intake. Identify areas for improvement and opportunities to align your nutrition with your goals.

Set Specific Goals: Clarify your goals related to body composition, performance, and overall health. Whether you're aiming to reduce body fat percentage, increase muscle mass, or improve energy levels, define specific, measurable objectives to guide your nutrition plan.

Calculate Your Macronutrient Needs: Determine your daily calorie requirements and macronutrient targets based on factors such as age, gender, weight, activity level, and goals. Online calculators and nutritional guidelines can provide a starting point for estimating your ideal macronutrient distribution.

Prioritize Whole, Nutrient-Dense Foods: Base your nutrition plan around whole, minimally processed foods rich in vitamins, minerals, fiber, and phytonutrients. Emphasize lean protein sources, complex carbohydrates, healthy fats, and an abundance of fruits and vegetables to support optimal health and body composition.

Plan Meals and Snacks: Create a meal plan that balances macronutrients, includes a variety of nutrient-dense foods, and accommodates your schedule and preferences. Aim for regular, balanced meals spaced throughout the day to maintain stable energy levels, support muscle recovery, and prevent excessive hunger.

Practice Portion Control: Pay attention to portion sizes and practice mindful eating to avoid overeating and promote satiety. Use visual cues, portion-control tools, and mindful eating practices such as chewing slowly and savoring each bite to regulate food intake and prevent mindless snacking.

Stay Flexible and Adaptable: While consistency is key to achieving long-term success, flexibility and adaptability are essential for maintaining adherence and sustainability. Allow for occasional indulgences, adjust your nutrition plan based on progress and feedback, and find a balance that works for your lifestyle and preferences.

By crafting a personalized nutrition plan that aligns with your goals, preferences, and lifestyle, you can optimize your dietary intake to support your journey to six-pack abs and overall health and wellness.

In Chapter 4, we'll explore effective workout strategies for sculpting the core, providing essential guidance on exercise selection, programming, and progression to maximize your abdominal development and enhance core strength and stability.

Chapter 4: Effective Workout Strategies

Achieving six-pack abs requires more than just targeting the abdominal muscles; it necessitates a holistic approach to fitness that encompasses strength training, cardiovascular exercise, and flexibility. In this chapter, we'll dispel the myth of spot reduction, emphasize the importance of a balanced workout routine, and provide guidance on targeting the core effectively through specific exercises.

4.1 The Myth of Spot Reduction: Debunking Misconceptions

Spot reduction refers to the belief that targeting specific areas of the body with exercise will result in localized fat loss. While it's tempting to believe that endless crunches or side bends will magically melt away belly fat, the reality is more nuanced. Here's why spot reduction is a myth:

Fat Loss Is Systemic: When the body metabolizes fat for energy, it does so in a systemic manner, drawing from fat stores throughout the body rather than selectively targeting specific areas. As a result, performing endless repetitions of abdominal exercises alone will not lead to significant fat loss in the abdominal region.

Genetics and Hormones Play a Role: Individual genetics and hormonal factors influence the distribution of body fat and the rate at which it is mobilized and burned. While some individuals may naturally store more fat in the abdominal area, others may carry excess fat in different areas of the body. Spot reduction cannot override these genetic predispositions.

Focus on Overall Fat Loss: Rather than fixating on spot reduction, focus on creating a caloric deficit through a combination of diet and exercise to promote overall fat loss. By reducing body fat percentage through consistent, balanced training and nutrition, you'll gradually reveal the underlying abdominal muscles and achieve visible abs.

By understanding the limitations of spot reduction and adopting a comprehensive approach to fitness, you can optimize your efforts and achieve sustainable results.

4.2 Building a Balanced Workout Routine: Incorporating Strength Training, Cardio, and Flexibility

A balanced workout routine is essential for achieving six-pack abs, enhancing overall fitness, and supporting long-term health and wellness. Incorporating a variety of training modalities ensures comprehensive development, improved performance, and reduced risk of injury. Here's how to structure a balanced workout routine:

Strength Training:

Prioritize compound exercises that engage multiple muscle groups simultaneously, such as squats, deadlifts, lunges, and presses, to maximize muscle activation and calorie expenditure.

Incorporate targeted core exercises that focus on the rectus abdominis, obliques, and lower back to strengthen and sculpt the abdominal muscles.

Gradually increase resistance and challenge your muscles through progressive overload to stimulate muscle growth and improve muscular definition.

Cardiovascular Exercise:

Include cardiovascular activities such as running, cycling, swimming, or high-intensity interval training (HIIT) to burn calories, improve cardiovascular health, and enhance fat loss.

Perform cardio workouts at varying intensities and durations to promote metabolic adaptation, prevent plateaus, and maintain motivation.

Incorporate both steady-state cardio and interval training to maximize calorie burn, improve endurance, and support overall fitness.

Flexibility and Mobility:

Incorporate dynamic warm-up exercises, foam rolling, and static stretching into your routine to improve flexibility, mobility, and joint range of motion.

Pay particular attention to stretching the muscles surrounding the core, including the hip flexors, hamstrings, and lower back, to alleviate tension and enhance movement quality.

Include yoga, Pilates, or mobility drills to promote core stability, balance, and body awareness, enhancing overall functional fitness.

By integrating strength training, cardiovascular exercise, and flexibility work into your workout routine, you'll create a comprehensive program that addresses all aspects of fitness and supports your quest for six-pack abs.

4.3 Targeting the Core: Exercises for Sculpting the Abs, Obliques, and Lower Back

Targeted core exercises are essential for sculpting the abdominal muscles, strengthening the obliques, and stabilizing the lower back. Incorporate the following exercises into your routine to effectively target the core:

Plank Variations: Planks are a cornerstone of core training, engaging the rectus abdominis, transverse abdominis, and erector spinae muscles. Experiment with standard planks, side planks, plank variations (e.g., plank with leg lifts, plank reaches), and plank progressions (e.g., weighted planks, stability ball planks) to challenge your core from different angles and intensities.

Crunch Variations: While traditional crunches primarily target the rectus abdominis, incorporating variations such as bicycle crunches, reverse crunches, and crunches on stability balls or exercise machines can provide additional stimulus and help sculpt the entire abdominal area.

Russian Twists: Russian twists target the obliques and improve rotational strength and stability. Perform them with a medicine ball, dumbbell, or bodyweight, rotating the torso from side to side while maintaining a stable, engaged core.

Leg Raises: Leg raises target the lower abdominals and hip flexors, helping to strengthen and define the lower portion of the abdominal wall. Perform lying leg raises, hanging leg raises, or captain's chair leg raises with controlled movement and emphasis on maintaining core stability.

Back Extensions: Back extensions strengthen the erector spinae muscles and promote spinal extension, contributing to overall core stability and lower back health. Perform back extensions on a hyperextension bench or stability ball, focusing on maintaining proper alignment and avoiding excessive arching of the lower back.

Incorporate these core exercises into your workout routine, progressively increasing intensity and difficulty over time to continue challenging your core muscles and promoting growth and definition.

By incorporating effective workout strategies, debunking misconceptions about spot reduction, and targeting the core through specific exercises, you'll lay the foundation for achieving six-pack abs and enhancing overall fitness and performance.

Chapter 6: Supplementing Your Efforts

In the pursuit of achieving your fitness goals, the incorporation of supplements can serve as valuable tools to complement your efforts. Understanding the role they play, identifying key supplements for specific objectives such as fat loss and muscle development, and being mindful of safety considerations are essential aspects to consider.

1. The Role of Supplements in Supporting Your Fitness Goals

Supplements serve as adjuncts to a well-rounded fitness regimen, aiming to optimize various aspects of performance, recovery, and overall health. While they are not substitutes for a balanced diet and consistent exercise routine, supplements can fill in nutritional gaps and provide targeted support where needed. By aiding in nutrient absorption, energy production, and muscle recovery, supplements can enhance the effectiveness of your fitness efforts.

2. Key Supplements for Enhancing Fat Loss and Muscle Development

a. Fat Loss:

Caffeine: Known for its thermogenic properties, caffeine can boost metabolism and increase fat oxidation, making it an effective supplement for supporting fat loss efforts.

Green Tea Extract: Rich in antioxidants and catechins, green tea extract promotes fat metabolism and may aid in weight management when combined with a healthy diet and exercise regimen.

L-Carnitine: Facilitating the transport of fatty acids into cells for energy production, L-carnitine supplementation can support fat utilization during exercise.

b. Muscle Development:

Whey Protein: As a fast-digesting protein source, whey protein is ideal for post-workout supplementation to promote muscle protein synthesis and facilitate muscle recovery.

Creatine: By increasing phosphocreatine stores in muscles, creatine supplementation enhances strength, power, and muscle mass gains during resistance training.

Branch Chain Amino Acids (BCAAs): Comprising essential amino acids like leucine, isoleucine, and valine, BCAA supplementation can aid in muscle repair, reduce muscle soreness, and support muscle growth.

3. Safety Considerations and Potential Risks Associated with Supplement Use

While supplements can offer benefits when used appropriately, it's crucial to approach their use with caution and awareness of potential risks. Consider the following safety considerations:

Quality and Purity: Choose supplements from reputable brands that undergo third-party testing to ensure quality and purity.

Dosage and Timing: Adhere to recommended dosages and timing guidelines provided by healthcare professionals or product labels to avoid adverse effects.

Interactions: Be mindful of potential interactions between supplements and medications you may be taking, and consult with a healthcare provider if necessary.

Transparency: Stay informed about the ingredients and formulations of supplements, and be wary of proprietary blends or undisclosed ingredients.

Individual Variability: Recognize that individual responses to supplements may vary, and what works well for one person may not yield the same results for another.

By approaching supplement use with knowledge, discernment, and moderation, you can maximize their benefits while minimizing potential risks, ultimately supporting your journey towards achieving your fitness goals.

Chapter 7: Overcoming Challenges

In the pursuit of six-pack abs and overall fitness, challenges are inevitable. From setbacks and plateaus to stress and self-doubt, navigating obstacles is an integral part of the journey. In this chapter, we'll explore strategies for overcoming common challenges, staying motivated, managing stress, and cultivating a resilient mindset for long-term success.

7.1 Dealing with Setbacks and Plateaus: Strategies for Staying Motivated

Setbacks and plateaus are common occurrences on the path to achieving six-pack abs. Whether it's a temporary lack of progress, an injury, or a deviation from your nutrition plan, setbacks can be discouraging. Here are strategies for staying motivated and overcoming setbacks:

Reframe Setbacks as Learning Opportunities: Instead of viewing setbacks as failures, see them as opportunities for growth and learning. Reflect on the factors that contributed to the setback and identify areas for improvement. Use setbacks as motivation to recommit to your goals and adjust your approach accordingly.

Focus on Progress, Not Perfection: Recognize that progress is rarely linear and that setbacks are a natural part of the journey. Celebrate small victories and milestones along the way, whether it's an increase in strength, a reduction in body fat percentage, or improved performance in your workouts. Embrace the process and trust that consistent effort will yield results over time.

Seek Support and Accountability: Lean on your support system—whether it's friends, family, or fellow fitness enthusiasts—for encouragement and accountability during challenging times. Share your goals and struggles with others who can offer support, guidance, and perspective. Accountability partners can help keep you motivated and accountable to your commitments.

Adjust Your Approach: If you've hit a plateau in your progress, it may be time to reassess your training, nutrition, and recovery strategies. Experiment with different workout routines, dietary approaches, or recovery techniques to break through plateaus and stimulate further progress. Stay open-minded and willing to adapt your approach based on feedback and results.

By adopting a proactive mindset, reframing setbacks as learning opportunities, and seeking support when needed, you can stay motivated and resilient in the face of challenges.

7.2 Managing Stress and Its Impact on Fitness Progress

Stress can have a significant impact on fitness progress, affecting everything from energy levels and motivation to recovery and performance. Here are strategies for managing stress and mitigating its impact on your fitness journey:

Prioritize Stress Management Techniques: Incorporate stress management techniques such as mindfulness meditation, deep breathing exercises, yoga, or relaxation techniques into your daily routine. These practices can help reduce stress hormones, promote relaxation, and improve overall well-being.

Maintain Work-Life Balance: Strive to maintain a healthy balance between work, fitness, and other aspects of your life. Avoid overcommitting yourself and prioritize activities that promote relaxation, enjoyment, and social connection. Setting boundaries and carving out time for self-care is essential for managing stress and preserving mental and emotional health.

Get Adequate Sleep: Prioritize quality sleep to support recovery, regulate stress hormones, and enhance overall resilience. Aim for 7-9 hours of uninterrupted sleep per night, and establish a consistent sleep schedule to optimize sleep quality and duration. Create a relaxing bedtime routine and minimize exposure to screens and stimulating activities before bedtime.

Practice Self-Compassion: Be kind to yourself during periods of stress or difficulty. Acknowledge your efforts and accomplishments, even if progress is slower than expected. Practice self-compassion by treating yourself with understanding, patience, and acceptance, especially during challenging times.

By managing stress effectively and prioritizing self-care, you can minimize its impact on your fitness progress and maintain a resilient mindset throughout your journey.

7.3 Cultivating a Resilient Mindset for Long-Term Success

Cultivating a resilient mindset is essential for long-term success in achieving six-pack abs and maintaining overall fitness and well-being. Here are strategies for developing resilience and navigating the ups and downs of your fitness journey:

Foster a Growth Mindset: Embrace challenges as opportunities for growth and learning, rather than insurmountable obstacles. Adopt a growth mindset that views setbacks and failures as temporary setbacks and opportunities to develop resilience, adaptability, and perseverance.

Focus on What You Can Control: Instead of fixating on external factors or circumstances beyond your control, focus on the aspects of your fitness journey that you can influence. Direct your energy and efforts toward setting and achieving actionable goals, making positive lifestyle changes, and maintaining consistency in your habits.

Practice Positive Self-Talk: Monitor your internal dialogue and challenge negative self-talk with affirmations, encouragement, and self-compassion. Cultivate a positive and empowering mindset by reframing setbacks as learning opportunities and focusing on your strengths and accomplishments.

Build a Supportive Community: Surround yourself with a supportive community of like-minded individuals who share your goals and values. Seek out positive role models, mentors, and accountability partners who can offer encouragement, guidance, and support during challenging times. Cultivate meaningful connections and draw strength from the collective wisdom and camaraderie of your community.

Embrace Resilience as a Skill: View resilience as a skill that can be developed and strengthened over time through practice and experience.

Embrace adversity as an opportunity to cultivate resilience muscles, build coping strategies, and enhance your ability to bounce back from setbacks with greater resilience and determination.

By cultivating a resilient mindset, managing stress effectively, and staying motivated in the face of challenges, you can navigate the complexities of your fitness journey with confidence, resilience, and perseverance.

Chapter 8: Lifestyle Integration

Integrating fitness into your daily life is essential for long-term success in achieving and maintaining six-pack abs and overall health and well-being. In this chapter, we'll explore the importance of recovery, including sleep, hydration, and stress management, as well as strategies for incorporating fitness into your daily routine and finding balance and enjoyment in the journey.

8.1 The Importance of Recovery: Sleep, Hydration, and Stress Management

Recovery is a critical component of any fitness regimen, facilitating muscle repair, hormone regulation, and overall recovery from physical exertion. Here's why prioritizing recovery is essential for optimizing your fitness journey:

Sleep: Adequate sleep is essential for physical and mental health, including muscle recovery, hormone regulation, and cognitive function. Aim for 7-9 hours of quality sleep per night, prioritizing consistency and creating a relaxing bedtime routine to support restful sleep.

Hydration: Proper hydration is crucial for optimal performance, nutrient delivery, and thermoregulation during exercise. Drink plenty of water throughout the day, especially before, during, and after workouts, to maintain hydration levels and support recovery.

Stress Management: Chronic stress can negatively impact recovery, performance, and overall well-being. Practice stress management techniques such as mindfulness meditation, deep breathing exercises, yoga, or progressive muscle relaxation to reduce stress hormones, promote relaxation, and improve resilience.

By prioritizing sleep, hydration, and stress management, you can enhance recovery, support your fitness goals, and optimize overall health and well-being.

8.2 Incorporating Fitness into Daily Life: Making Sustainable Lifestyle Changes

Incorporating fitness into your daily life requires making sustainable lifestyle changes that align with your goals, preferences, and priorities. Here are strategies for integrating fitness seamlessly into your daily routine:

Schedule Regular Workouts: Treat exercise like any other appointment or commitment by scheduling regular workouts into your calendar. Choose a time of day that works best for you and stick to a consistent exercise routine to build momentum and establish a habit.

Find Activities You Enjoy: Explore different types of physical activity to find activities you genuinely enjoy and look forward to. Whether it's hiking, cycling, dancing, or playing a team sport, choose activities that align with your interests and bring you joy.

Incorporate Movement Throughout the Day: Look for opportunities to incorporate movement into your daily routine, such as taking the stairs instead of the elevator, walking or biking to work, or stretching during breaks at work. Every bit of movement adds up and contributes to your overall activity level.

Make Healthy Food Choices: Support your fitness goals by making nutritious food choices that fuel your body and support recovery. Prioritize whole, minimally processed foods rich in lean protein, complex carbohydrates, healthy fats, fruits, and vegetables.

Practice Active Recreation: Instead of sedentary activities like watching TV or scrolling through social media, engage in active recreation that promotes movement and physical activity. Explore outdoor activities, hobbies, or recreational sports that keep you active and engaged.

Create a Supportive Environment: Surround yourself with a supportive environment that reinforces your fitness goals and encourages healthy behaviors. Seek out friends, family members, or fitness communities who share your values and support your journey.

By making sustainable lifestyle changes and integrating fitness into your daily routine, you can establish habits that support your long-term health, fitness, and well-being.

8.3 Finding Balance and Enjoying the Journey

While achieving six-pack abs is a worthy goal, it's essential to find balance and enjoyment in the journey. Here's how to maintain balance and perspective while pursuing your fitness goals:

Set Realistic Expectations: Recognize that progress takes time and that setbacks and plateaus are a natural part of the journey. Set realistic expectations, celebrate small victories, and be patient with yourself as you work toward your goals.

Practice Self-Compassion: Be kind to yourself during challenging times, and practice self-compassion by treating yourself with understanding, patience, and acceptance. Focus on progress, not perfection, and celebrate your efforts and accomplishments along the way.

Embrace Variety and Exploration: Keep your fitness journey exciting and engaging by exploring new activities, trying different workouts, and challenging yourself in new ways. Embrace variety in your routine and be open to experimenting with different approaches to fitness.

Prioritize Enjoyment: Find activities and workouts that bring you joy and satisfaction, and prioritize enjoyment in your fitness journey. Whether it's dancing, hiking, lifting weights, or practicing yoga, choose activities that make you feel good and align with your interests and preferences.

Focus on Non-Aesthetic Benefits: While six-pack abs may be a desirable outcome, focus on the non-aesthetic benefits of fitness, such as improved energy levels, mood, confidence, and overall health and well-being. Shift your focus from appearance to how you feel and function in your daily life.

Practice Gratitude: Cultivate a sense of gratitude for your body's abilities, the support of others, and the opportunities for growth and self-improvement. Express gratitude for the progress you've made.

Chapter 9: Navigating Plateaus and Adjustments

Plateaus are common occurrences in any fitness journey, including the quest for six-pack abs. Recognizing signs of plateau and knowing when to adjust your approach are crucial for overcoming stagnation and continuing to make progress. In this chapter, we'll explore strategies for identifying plateaus, making adjustments to your workout routine and nutrition plan, and the role of rest and recovery in breaking through plateaus.

9.1 Identifying Signs of Plateau and When to Change Your Approach

Plateaus occur when your progress stalls despite consistent effort in your workouts and nutrition plan. Recognizing signs of plateau allows you to take proactive steps to adjust your approach and stimulate further progress. Here are common signs of plateau and indicators that it may be time to change your approach:

Stalled Progress: If you've stopped seeing improvements in muscle definition, strength gains, or reductions in body fat percentage despite consistent effort, you may have hit a plateau.

Lack of Motivation: A decline in motivation or enthusiasm for your workouts may indicate that you've reached a plateau. If you're feeling bored, uninspired, or unmotivated by your current routine, it may be time for a change.

Decreased Performance: A decline in performance during workouts, such as decreased strength, endurance, or workout intensity, can be a sign of plateau. If you're struggling to complete workouts or feeling fatigued more quickly than usual, it may be a sign that your body needs a new stimulus.

Persistent Fatigue or Soreness: Experiencing persistent fatigue, soreness, or muscle stiffness despite adequate rest and recovery may indicate that your body is not adapting to your current training regimen.

When you notice signs of plateau, it's essential to evaluate your current approach and make adjustments to stimulate further progress.

9.2 Adjusting Your Workout Routine and Nutrition Plan for Continued Progress

Making adjustments to your workout routine and nutrition plan is essential for overcoming plateaus and continuing to make progress toward your fitness goals. Here are strategies for adjusting your approach:

Change Up Your Workouts: Modify your workout routine by incorporating new exercises, changing the order of exercises, adjusting sets and reps, or increasing resistance to provide a new stimulus to your muscles. Experiment with different training modalities such as circuit training, interval training, or functional training to challenge your body in new ways.

Progressive Overload: Gradually increase the intensity, volume, or complexity of your workouts to continue challenging your muscles and stimulating growth. Incorporate progressive overload principles by increasing weight, reps, or sets over time to promote muscle adaptation and prevent plateau.

Periodization: Implement periodization techniques such as linear periodization, undulating periodization, or block periodization to vary training variables and optimize performance while minimizing the risk of plateau. Periodization allows you to cycle through phases of different intensities, volumes, and training focuses to prevent stagnation and promote continual progress.

Nutrition Adjustments: Evaluate your nutrition plan and make adjustments to support your fitness goals. Consider adjusting your calorie intake, macronutrient ratios, meal timing, or supplementation based on changes in activity level, metabolism, or goals. Consult with a registered dietitian or nutritionist for personalized guidance and recommendations.

By making strategic adjustments to your workout routine and nutrition plan, you can break through plateaus and continue making progress toward your fitness goals.

9.3 The Role of Rest and Recovery in Breaking Through Plateaus

Rest and recovery play a crucial role in breaking through plateaus and optimizing performance. Here's how prioritizing rest and recovery can help you overcome stagnation and make progress:

Active Recovery: Incorporate active recovery strategies such as light cardio, stretching, foam rolling, or yoga into your routine to promote blood flow, reduce muscle soreness, and enhance recovery between workouts. Active recovery helps alleviate fatigue and stiffness while promoting relaxation and mental well-being.

Deload Weeks: Implement deload weeks or periods of reduced training volume or intensity to allow your body to recover and adapt to previous training stimuli. Deload weeks prevent overtraining, reduce the risk of injury, and promote long-term progress by facilitating recovery and minimizing fatigue.

Quality Sleep: Prioritize quality sleep to support recovery, hormone regulation, and overall well-being. Aim for 7-9 hours of uninterrupted sleep per night, and create a relaxing sleep environment conducive to restful sleep. Quality sleep is essential for muscle repair, cognitive function, and immune health.

Nutrition for Recovery: Optimize your nutrition plan to support recovery by consuming adequate calories, protein, carbohydrates, and micronutrients to replenish glycogen stores, repair muscle tissue, and support immune function. Focus on nutrient-dense foods that provide essential vitamins, minerals, and antioxidants to promote recovery and reduce inflammation.

By prioritizing rest and recovery, you can optimize your body's ability to adapt to training stimuli, break through plateaus, and continue making progress toward your fitness goals.

In Chapter 10, we'll explore strategies for sustaining long-term success and maintaining your six-pack abs for life, including tips for consistency, accountability, and lifestyle integration.

Chapter 10: Celebrating Success and Sustaining Progress

After putting in the hard work and dedication to achieve your six-pack abs, it's essential to celebrate your success and implement strategies for sustaining your progress in the long term. In this chapter, we'll explore ways to recognize milestones, maintain your hard-earned results, and embrace fitness as a lifelong journey.

10.1 Recognizing Milestones and Celebrating Achievements

As you progress on your fitness journey, it's important to acknowledge and celebrate the milestones and achievements along the way. Celebrating success not only boosts motivation and confidence but also reinforces positive behaviors and helps maintain momentum. Here are some ways to recognize milestones and celebrate achievements:

Set Milestone Goals: Break down your overarching fitness goals into smaller, achievable milestones or checkpoints. Whether it's reaching a certain body fat percentage, achieving a new personal best in

the gym, or mastering a challenging exercise,
set specific goals that you can work towards
and celebrate once achieved.

Track Progress: Keep track of your progress
using methods such as before-and-after
photos, body measurements, strength gains, or
workout logs. Regularly review your progress
to see how far you've come and celebrate the
improvements you've made along the way.

Reward Yourself: Treat yourself to non-food
rewards or experiences as a way to celebrate
your achievements. Whether it's buying a new
workout outfit, booking a massage, or planning
a fun activity with friends, choose rewards that
align with your values and reinforce your
commitment to your goals.

Share Your Success: Share your achievements
with friends, family, or your fitness community

to celebrate your progress and receive encouragement and support. Celebrating success with others not only enhances your sense of accomplishment but also strengthens your support network and accountability.

By recognizing milestones and celebrating achievements, you can stay motivated and inspired on your fitness journey.

10.2 Strategies for Maintaining Your Hard-Earned Results

Maintaining your hard-earned results requires ongoing commitment, consistency, and a balanced approach to fitness and nutrition.

Here are strategies for sustaining your progress in the long term:

Prioritize Consistency: Consistency is key to maintaining your results over time. Continue to follow a balanced workout routine and nutritious diet, making exercise and healthy eating habits a non-negotiable part of your lifestyle.

Set New Goals: Once you've achieved your initial goals, set new challenges and objectives to keep yourself motivated and engaged. Whether it's improving strength, mastering new skills, or trying new activities, setting new goals helps maintain focus and momentum.

Focus on Maintenance: Shift your mindset from constantly striving for progress to focusing on maintenance and sustainability. Rather than always pushing for new personal bests or chasing aesthetic goals, prioritize maintaining your current level of fitness, health, and well-being.

Be Flexible: Allow for flexibility in your routine and approach to fitness, recognizing that life may throw curveballs or unexpected challenges. Adapt your workouts, nutrition plan, and schedule as needed to accommodate changes in circumstances or priorities while staying true to your long-term goals.

Monitor Progress: Continuously monitor your progress and make adjustments as needed to ensure you're staying on track. Regularly assess your workouts, nutrition, and lifestyle habits to identify areas for improvement and course corrections.

Practice Self-Compassion: Be kind to yourself and practice self-compassion when setbacks or challenges arise. Remember that progress is not always linear, and it's okay to have ups and downs along the way. Treat yourself with the same kindness and understanding you would offer to a friend facing similar circumstances.

By implementing these strategies, you can sustain your hard-earned results and continue to progress on your fitness journey for the long term.

10.3 Embracing Fitness as a Lifelong Journey

Finally, it's important to recognize that fitness is not just about achieving a specific goal but rather embracing it as a lifelong journey. Embrace the process of continual growth, learning, and self-improvement, and enjoy the journey as much as the destination. Here's how to embrace fitness as a lifelong journey:

Cultivate a Growth Mindset: Adopt a growth mindset that views fitness as a journey of self-discovery and personal development. Embrace challenges, setbacks, and failures as opportunities for growth and learning rather than obstacles to overcome.

Focus on Overall Well-Being: Shift your focus from solely aesthetic goals to prioritize overall health, well-being, and quality of life. Seek to cultivate habits and behaviors that promote physical, mental, and emotional wellness, rather than solely focusing on external markers of success.

Find Joy in Movement: Explore different forms of physical activity and exercise that bring you joy, fulfillment, and satisfaction. Whether it's hiking in nature, dancing to your favorite music, or practicing yoga, find activities that nourish your body, mind, and soul.

Build a Supportive Community: Surround yourself with a supportive community of like-minded individuals who share your values and support your journey. Connect with friends, family, or fitness communities who inspire and motivate you to be your best self.

Practice Gratitude: Cultivate a sense of gratitude for your body's capabilities, the opportunity to pursue fitness goals, and the support of others along the way. Express gratitude for the journey itself, recognizing that every step forward is a gift to be cherished.

By embracing fitness as a lifelong journey, you can cultivate a positive and sustainable approach to health and well-being that extends far beyond achieving six-pack abs.

In Conclusion, celebrating success, sustaining progress, and embracing fitness as a lifelong journey are essential components of achieving and maintaining six-pack abs and overall health and well-being. By recognizing milestones, staying committed to your goals, and enjoying the process, you can cultivate a fulfilling and sustainable approach to fitness that enriches your life in countless ways.

www.ingramcontent.com/pod-product-compliance
Lightning Source LLC
Chambersburg PA
CBHW050817250726
48653CB00006B/2281